There's No Money in Dead People

Advice from a nurse on how to ensure the end-of-life care you want

By Traci Annette Powell, CNP

Dedication...

To my husband Paul and my daughters Jazzma, Chelza, and Asti...

Thank you for forgiving me of all my faults, and still loving me in spite of them.

Please remember:

I am a nurse, not an author. ☺

This is a self-published book. I did not have an editor, a major publishing company, or a marketing department.

I do believe I have something important to share. It is my hope you will overlook my novice attempt at writing in exchange for some information which may be beneficial to you.

TABLE OF CONTENTS

INTRODUCTION

The title of this book came from the sick sense of humor that only a person who works in medicine could really appreciate. After watching patient after patient who were either terminally ill, brain dead, or at the end of life due to chronic illness and advanced age, be given aggressive treatment after aggressive treatment, one procedure after another, lab tests followed by more lab tests, etc, etc, etc, with everyone knowing the patient wasn't going to survive, those infamous words came out of my mouth one night when one of my co-workers asked "Why are we doing this?" ...I sarcastically replied "Because there's no money in dead people."

Now for the record: I understand and know personally how difficult it is to lose someone you love. Letting go is never easy.

I also have the utmost respect for physicians. Most doctors are certainly not in medicine for the money. God knows they could have made more money with better hours and lots less headaches if they would have chosen to be an accountant, lawyer or engineer. Even after all these years I am still amazed by physicians.

I've seen them work 16+ hour days and then get awaken several times throughout the night with calls from the hospital or their patients. They get up the next day and do it again…and again…and again. I've seen doctors who have practiced for twenty or thirty years who still get upset when one of their patients die or they have to tell a young mother she's lost her pregnancy (Thanks Dr Orth).

So my intentions are not to offend anyone but rather to give the public an inside look at how things sometimes work in healthcare and make suggestions as to how they might be able to ensure their wishes are honored in regards to their end-of-life care.

Most of us have a pretty good idea about how we want to die: at home, at peace, quickly, with family, without pain. And at a ripe old age.

But progress begets paradox: We've gotten so good at the last goal, it swallowed the others, so we live longer but die slower.

From TIME article, May 5, 2008 by Nancy Gibbs

Hi!

My name is Traci Powell and I am a family nurse practitioner. My interest in 'Do Not Resuscitate' orders originated while working as a critical care nurse, spending time in both an emergency department and an intensive care unit. Until I started working in critical care I had no idea how useless DNR (Do Not Resuscitate) orders were, even though I had worked in healthcare for over twenty years. So I got to thinking….if I worked for years in the medical field and was unaware of how things REALLY worked, then what chance does a person with no medical background have when they are faced with one of the most stressful times of their lives?!

..And so began my journey as an author.

Let me begin by sharing with you a couple true stories which started my interest in DNR orders…

At 92 she just wanted left alone…

One night I had to start an IV on an elderly lady who had a fractured hip and was going to surgery the next day. She was ninety-two years old, blind, and weighed about eighty pounds. Every time I took her hand to try and start the IV, she would pull away from me and say in her little weak voice "PLEASE just leave me alone". I stopped what I was doing and went out and told the charge nurse what the patient was saying. I told her obviously the woman did not want all this treatment and surgery done. The charge nurse looked at me and sighed, then said, "But the family wants everything done." And so the little old lady, at the age of 92, went off to surgery the next day.

He had been through enough…

One evening while working in ICU a middle aged man with advanced multiple sclerosis was in the emergency room getting ready to be transferred up to our unit.

When I got report from the ER nurse she told me the man was in respiratory distress, close to respiratory failure, but he had repeatedly told the ER staff he did not want intubated and put on the ventilator. He was brought up to me with respirations in the 40s and 50s. He was obviously in significant respiratory distress but still very much alert and oriented. I explained to him that unless his respiratory status started improving, he would soon go apnic and stop breathing. I asked him three times "If you stop breathing, do you want us to put a tube down your throat to help you breath?" Each time he clearly and firmly said "No". I then asked him if his heart stopped, did he want us to do CPR which would entail doing chest compressions. After a few seconds of thought, he said yes, that would be o.k. I then asked him again about the ventilator and he adamantly replied that he did not want on a ventilator.

After getting the patient settled into the unit I allowed the family back into the room and reviewed with them what the patient's wishes were. The wife and sons stated that he had had a long battle with MS and that he had been all over the country for treatment. They also stated the patient had been on a ventilator many times in the past. The family then told me they wanted him to be resuscitated if needed, including intubation and placing him on a ventilator. I explained to the family that he was alert and oriented and that he had the right to choose what treatments he wanted and which ones he did not. The wife looked at me and said "I am his POA (power of attorney) and as soon as he goes unconscious I'm going to tell you to intubate him." It was close to the end of my shift and when she told me that I said a prayer. I prayed 'God please do not let this gentleman code until I am off the clock', because I honestly did not know what I would do. I knew what the man's wishes were. He had been through a lot, he knew what it was like to be on a ventilator and didn't want back on one, and he had a terminal illness. I also knew what the law said--once incapacitated, your POA can legally make your healthcare decisions for you. If you do not have a POA, then your next of kin makes the decisions, beginning with your spouse. The Lord answered my prayers. My shift ended and seven minutes later as I was walking out the door, the man went into respiratory failure, stopped breathing, and the wife told the staff to intubate him. And they did.

Another DNR order missed...

One day we received a patient in ICU who had come into the Emergency Department by squad who was in full arrest (no breathing, no heart beat). The

Emergency Department staff successfully resuscitated the patient and sent her up to us on a ventilator. When the family got to the hospital, they were furious. The patient had a DNR order. She did not want CPR done; she did not want on a ventilator. We discontinued the IVs and ventilator and the patient died.

Fact: Fifty percent of all elderly people who break a hip will die within one year.

FIFTY PERCENT.....50%

They don't die from the hip fracture; or from the surgical repair of the hip; they die from loss of mobility. While the body is immobile, other systems start to fail like the lungs, the heart, and the kidneys. So when President Obama made the comment after the death of his beloved grandmother about whether giving people "a hip replacement when they're terminally ill is a sustainable model", he was right in his thinking.

In case you haven't noticed, in the medical field we have our own language. We use words that most people have never heard before. Many of us in medicine have been in this field for so long that we forget that other people outside of healthcare have absolutely no idea what we're talking about. Occasionally you will run across the arrogant medical professional who just likes to throw out big words to show off and try to impress you. Ignore those people. One of my goals for this book is to explain to people who have no medical background what some of these terms mean. Let's first review each type of code status:

Types of Code Statuses

- **Full Code**: Everything is done

- **DNR-CCA**: Everything is done up until cardiac arrest or respiratory arrest

- **DNR – CC**: Comfort care only

Now let's take a closer look at what each code statue means.

A **full code** is what you are if you don't have a DNR order. Unfortunately, this is the category where most of us fall. You could have CPR (cardiopulmonary resuscitation), be intubated and placed on a ventilator (machine that breaths for you), receive nutrition through an IV or an NG tube (nasogastric-tube means tube down nose into stomach), have cardiac (heart) IV drips to raise or lower your blood pressure, and have labs, x-rays, and procedures done. Basically everything but the kitchen sink.

A **DNR-CCA** includes doing everything up until the heart stops beating or you go into respiratory failure (stop breathing). This code status includes things like lab tests, procedures, cardiac drips, oral medications, and nutrition. We will not do chest compressions or intubate you. The only problem with this is that most of us in healthcare will not stand by and let you go into respiratory failure. Once we see you getting into respiratory distress, we'll sedate you, intubate you, and put you on a ventilator. And this is fine in many cases. Some patients simply need a couple days to get the lungs cleared out or to give the body a break from expending a lot of energy on working to breath.

While we're talking of intubation, let me explain what that means. Intubation means putting a tube, called an endotracheal tube, down your throat and placing you on a ventilator. Some people will choose to add on a "No intubation" order with their code status.

A **DNR-CC** order means to provide comfort care and allow natural death. For a patient with a DNR-CC order, we will provide things like liberal pain medication, positioning, suctioning of the airway, and oxygen. Anything that would make the patient more comfortable.

Please note: When chest compressions are done during CPR, your sternum and/or ribs are often broke. That is how much force we have to use to pump your heart efficiently enough to get the oxygen-carrying blood to your vital organs...most notable, the brain. CPR is a tool that can save lives and I believe everyone should be taught how to perform CPR; however, the public does not realize how small the survival rate is when CPR is performed. For out of hospital cardiac arrest, survival at one year is 2% with standard CPR and 5% with use of an AED (automatic external defibrillator). Researchers found that even when cardiac arrests take place with medical help right at hand, only 22% of patients live to return home from the hospital. One in seven can no longer live independently because of the long-term damage. Ruth, an ICU nurse I used to work with, gave me this great T-shirt once that said:

<u>C</u>ompassion – <u>P</u>ersonal Choice – <u>R</u>espect

DNR

Unless you witnessed my cardiac arrest, caught my body as it fell, and did immediate, picture perfect CPR while you set up a bi-phasic defibrillator which discharged 200 joules into my heart within 60 seconds of the arrest, and have appropriate drugs standing by, within arms reach…

DON'T TOUCH ME!

This is not meant to discourage you, only to help you have a reasonable expectation of what resuscitation can and cannot do. If you have a child or young, healthy adult who is a victim of drowning, for instance, prompt and correctly performed CPR is very successful in resuscitating these folks.

Now let's start going over some of the reasons why DNR orders frequently don't work. While researching the literature for why these DNR orders fail so often, I identified ten major problems:

1. Lack of clear communication

2. Multiple physicians on a case with different opinions

3. No one wants to be the bearer of bad news

4. Families are just not ready

5. Time issues verses point of no return

6. Surrogate's guilt in making decision/signing DNR orders

7. DNR papers are not available

8. Difficulty in understanding DNR orders

9. Financial benefits to families

10. Religious/moral beliefs of families and physicians

Problem #1: Lack of Clear Communication

Typical scenario: Elderly patient has had a myocardial infarction (heart attack), had to be resuscitated, is on a ventilator for full respiratory support, and has cardiac drips keeping his blood pressure up. After several days like this a physician comes into the room and tells the family "I think he's turning the corner." What he means is the guy's labs are getting better. What the family thinks is that dad is going to be o.k. and get to go home in a couple days and be just like he was before he came into the hospital…**Wrong**.

With damage to the brain stem (this is very bad), a person will do what is called 'posturing'. They will either decorticate or decerebrate, depending on where the damage is and how bad it is. With decorticate, a patient will turn their hands and arms inward toward their body and stiffen their legs out. With decerebrate, a patient will turn their hands and arms outward and stiffen their legs. Even when families are told the patient is brain dead, when they see their loved one doing this posturing, they will say "Look, she's squeezing my hand" or "When I talk to her, she's responding to me and grabbing my hand"…**Wrong**.

Patients and their families don't understand the medical terminology. It is very confusing. I compare medical terminology to trying to read legal documents or an insurance policy. Research has shown that families want doctors and nurses to be frank and not avoid talking about bad news. Each time I'm in a room with a patient who is posturing and a family member says "Look, she's squeezing my hand!" I explain to them what posturing is and that it is not the patient voluntarily responding to them. I've had family members say they wondered deep down if that was what was really happening and I've had others say "I don't care what you say, I know mom's responding to me." All we can do as healthcare professionals is give the families factual information in a compassionate manner and in terminology they can understand.

There are those-soldiers and nurses, poets and priests-

for whom death is a sure companion. But most people

treat it as a notorious celebrity watched from afar,

fascinated but removed, until they have no choice,

preferring myth to truth

From TIME article, May 5, 2008 by Nancy Gibbs

Problem #2: Multiple Providers on Case with Different Opinions

A typical patient in an intensive care unit can easily have five or six different physicians managing their case. They usually have a cardiologist (heart doc), a nephrologist (kidney doc), pulmonologist (lung doc), and an internist or family physician for overall medical management. Depending on what you are in the hospital for, you could also have an infectious disease specialist or a neurologist (brain doc) involved in your care.

Have you ever tried to get a group of people to agree on one thing? It's next to impossible isn't it? This is why jury trials are so popular with criminals! It is no different in medicine. The pulmonologist may think the patient is doing great…from his view of looking at the patient's respiratory status. The nephrologist sees the patient going downhill because his kidneys are failing and he will soon need to be on dialysis in order to live. And the cardiologist thinks there really isn't anything else we can do for the man because his heart is big and floppy and can't pump the blood efficiently anymore. We've got him on three different cardiac drips trying to keep a blood pressure and he only has an ejection fraction of 15% (this is bad). The problem here is each provider will go in and tell the patient and their family what their opinion is on how the patient is doing. I've seen five different doctors go into a room, one at a time throughout the day, and the first four docs will tell the family "It doesn't look good. I don't think he's going to pull out of this." Then the fifth doc goes in and says "He's starting to look better." But remember, the patient is only looking better from this specialist's view, perhaps from a respiratory status. It still doesn't mean his heart is going to improve or his kidneys are not going to shut down. But when it comes to someone we love, at the end of the day, we will "hear" only the optimistic voice. The one that said "He's starting to look better."

I have seen many families 'fire' physicians off of their loved ones case because of this type of situation. They will say 'That doctor said he was going to die but doctor so and so said he was getting better.' You need to remember that when a specialist gives you a report or opinion, they are usually telling you how that specific part of the body is doing-the lung, the heart, whatever. Just because

one part of the body is doing well doesn't mean mom is going to go home in a

couple days and be her old self again. **Look at the whole picture!**

Problem #3: No One Wants to be the Bearer of Bad News

Despite the growing emphasis on end-of-life care, neither physicians nor nurses think their educational preparation or clinical experiences have prepared them well to help patients and patient's families at the end of life. O.K. Go back and read that last sentence again. It is very true.

I hope you are sitting down because I have some earth shattering news...are you ready?......nurses and doctors are human beings just like you. We get tired, we make mistakes, and we don't like to give people bad news. Many nights when I would get home from work my husband would ask me how my day was. Often the best reply I could give him was "Well, no one died today." That translated into 'It was a hard day'.

Most of us in healthcare go into the field because we REALLY like helping people. God knows it isn't because of the good hours, short educational requirements, or pleasant surroundings. I doubt there is a doctor or nurse anywhere who gets up in the morning and says to their self "Gee, I hope I get to tell someone today that the person they have loved for the last fifty years is going to die soon."

In my research I found that many nurses reported learning to provide care for patients at the end of life by "trial and error". That's usually never a good way to learn anything. Our nursing and medical schools need a requirement in their educational curriculum on how to talk with patients and families about death and dying. We could use nurses who work in palliative and hospice care to teach it. I've seen those nurses at work and they are simply amazing.

Problem #4: Families are Just Not Ready

This is especially true when a person becomes critically ill or injured unexpectedly. I think just about every family has one member who has a falling out with the others and they go for years not speaking or just having minimal contact. And then mom or dad become comatose from a stroke and is on full life support. The recommendation is to discontinue life support and allow natural death. But here comes the 'black sheep' of the family who now realizes they may never be able to make amends with their parent and so they adamantly fight the other family members in stopping life support. Here is the problem: The law says healthcare workers can follow a DNR order and will not be held liable for the patient's death. That doesn't mean a family member will still not sue. Even though you know you are legally correct and would win the lawsuit, it costs thousands and thousands of dollars to go to court. Not to mention the huge mental and emotional toll it takes on a physician. So when that 'black sheep' says "I'm going to sue you if you take mom off life support", most of the time, we leave her on.

Another instance where families have a hard time letting go is when there is an important date approaching. Let me share with you another true story:

We had a frail, elderly woman in our ICU who required everything we had to keep her alive. It was obvious that she was not going to get better. Every day we would talk to her husband about discontinuing all the machines and drips and allowing her to die. It was painful for us nurses to take care of the lady because we knew all the things we were doing to her was causing her pain. Her husband would never really respond to us when we would explain to him how bad her condition was. He would come early every morning and stay at her bedside all day. At the end of each day he would go to leave, saying that he would be back the next morning. This went on for over a week. I became frustrated with the husband. I thought to myself, how can you let someone you love so much suffer like this lady was. Then one day he said to me "You know, on Thursday it will be our 51st wedding anniversary." Now it made sense. He wanted to share one more anniversary with her. She lived until Thursday and they got to spend their 51st

anniversary together. The next day the husband told us to discontinue all the life

support. We did and the lady died within minutes.

Problem #5: Time Issue verses Point of No Return

Usually a person can only be on a ventilator with an endotracheal tube in for about two weeks. After that a decision has to be made as to whether to terminally extubate (take the patient off the vent and allow natural death) or to put a tracheotomy (a small tube placed in a hole made in the throat) in the patient. Often when a tracheotomy tube is placed, many patients will also have a peg tube (a tube placed in a hole made in the stomach for feeding) inserted at the same time. Here's the problem: Once you have a trach and a peg tube, you're stuck. You have a permanent airway and a route for nutrition. So you can breath and you can be fed…for a very, very long time.

It is true that many people just need more time to recover from their illness or injury. Lots of people have had a tracheotomy and a peg tube reversed and went on to live very happy and productive lives. Many times these are wonderful, life-saving procedures. What you have to look at though is the whole picture of the person's health. If the person is in their eighties, has COPD (chronic obstructive pulmonary disease), CHF (congestive heart failure), and chronic renal (kidney) failure, what are the chances of that person ever getting off the vent or having that trach reversed?

I have never seen a person terminally extubated from a ventilator who had a tracheotomy. If you are terminally extubated from the ventilator with an endotracheal tube in place, the tube is removed from your throat. It is a significant procedure to put that tube back down your throat to put you back on the ventilator. If you have a tracheotomy however, you simply pop the ventilator off and on the tracheotomy opening. It's very simple. So what happens to these elderly people with multiple chronic illnesses who can't get off the ventilator? They often get sent to a long term rehabilitation center where they get turned every two hours for the next ten years. Why? Because again, you have a permanent airway and a way to feed them, which keeps them alive.

The research shows that many families say later they wish they hadn't allowed a tracheotomy, or that the patient never would have wanted a tracheotomy.

Problem #6: Surrogate's Guilt in Making Decision/Signing DNR Orders

Unfortunately the majority of 'Do Not Resuscitate' orders are authorized by surrogates, not the patient. The research shows that many patients who lack capacity at the time of the DNR decision making were able to do so just two weeks earlier.

Some of the comments from husbands, wives, and children who have signed DNR orders…

"I felt guilty if I didn't because she would suffer; I felt guilty if I did because she would die"

"I feel like I'm signing his death warrent."

If you do not have a DNR order, the law says your spouse is authorized to make the decision for you. If you do not have a spouse, then it's your oldest child (of legal age). If there are no children then it is up to your parent. And the list works its way on through the family. I have seen DNR decisions made by distant cousins, family friends, and social workers. This often happens when a person is very old and has outlived the other family members.

Problem #7: DNR Papers Are Not Available

It is very difficult to know in many situations whether or not a patient has a DNR order. Let me give you a couple examples.

- A patient comes into the emergency department by squad with no family and unable to communicate.

- A nursing home sends an elderly, confused patient to the emergency department without their DNR orders.

- A person is out at the mall doing their daily walking exercise and has a massive heart attack. Many people know CPR and AEDs (automatic external defibrillator) are now more readily available. These devices are often kept at schools, malls, airports, just about any place that attracts large numbers of people. Most of us don't normally keep our DNR papers on us at all times, so the Good Samaritan starts CPR on you and zaps you with the AED!

One of my favorite stories involves a retired ICU nurse who knows very well how things really work in medicine. Not only did she have all the proper paperwork filled out for a DNR order and a living will, along with making sure her family were very much aware of and supportive of her wishes, but she even went to a tattoo parlor and had "DO NOT RUSUSCITATE" tattooed on her chest!

Smart woman.

Barrier #8: Difficulty in Understanding DNR Orders

The DNR order came into being in the United States in the 1960s. For a DNR order to be valid there may be rules such as the use of a special form and/or additional signatures of a doctor and /or witnesses. These requirements vary widely from state to state.

In Maryland, for example, only state DNR orders are acceptable, and they require much verification, witnesses and doctor's signatures in order to be valid. Virginia, on the other hand, allows patients to receive a DNR order with relative ease and will accept them from most jurisdictions.

After all these years in the healthcare field, I still have trouble understanding them. In fact, there are many nurses and doctors who do not understand the difference between a DNR-CCA and a DNR-CC. DNR orders are not clear and they can be interrupted in different ways. For instance, there is debate among healthcare providers regarding whether administering oxygen to a person with a DNR-CC is providing comfort or simply prolonging life.

Here's another real-life story for you:

In the ICU where I worked we had a patient tracking board with the last names of the patients, their room number, their admitting doctor, and which nurse was caring for that patient for the current shift. Beside each name we would write if they were a DNR-CCA or a DNR-CC. There was no special notation if they were a full code. Occasionally we would have a patient who would be a DNR-CCA plus 'no intubation'. (Now remember you're not suppose to be intubated with respiratory failure if you are a DNR-CCA but we don't stand around and let you go into failure; we intubate you when you get into distress). So our little system works out pretty good most of the time. We can quickly see what each patient's code status is with a glance at the board.

One day I walk into work and see a note on the board by one man's name that said "A couple chest compressions o.k." I asked what this was all about and apparently when the gentleman came in the night before they asked him what his code status was and he didn't have any. So they explained to him what each code status meant and asked him if he wanted a code status other than 'full code'. He said he 'guessed it would be o.k.' to put a tube down his throat if needed but he would only want "a couple chest compressions done". The admitting nurse tried her best to explain to him that what he was wanting really wasn't feasible, but the man was set on wanting CPR if needed but only with just a couple compressions.

Each time I took care of that patient I would say a little prayer, "Please don't let him code on my shift." I mean, what the hell was I going to do with that code status?! I could just picture it in my mind: He goes into arrest; I hit the 'code' button to call the team in; I do "a couple chest compressions"; look to see if he's back or not; he's not. The whole code team consisting of an ED physician, any other physicians on the unit at that time, the pharmacist, the respiratory therapist, the lab personnel, the x-ray technician , and several other ICU nurses- all run into the room and there I stand announcing: "It's o.k. I've already ran the entire code. He didn't make it so you can all leave now." Give me a break! But this is the kind of thing that happens all the time. People don't understand what goes on during a code. And so the reason for this book. By the way, the little guy did not code (Thank God!) and was moved out of the unit within a few days.

Progress is being made in some states regarding development of easier to understand DNR orders. Some states are now using advance directives called POLST and MOLST. POLST stands for 'Physician orders for Life-Sustaining Treatment' and MOLST stands for 'Medical Orders for Life-Sustaining Treatment'. The difference between the two is that POLSTs have to be signed by a physician and MOLSTs allow for nurse practitioners (NP) and physician assistants (PA) to also sign off on these orders. YEA! Maybe I'm being biased but I believe there is a huge advantage for people living in states who use MOLSTs. I can't speak for PAs but I know for a fact that NPs are much more likely to address a patient and/or family about end-of-life care.

What makes the MOLSTs and POLSTs nicer than the DNR orders is that they address very specifically what a person wants. These orders usually consist of sections regarding:

- CPR or no CPR

- Intubation or no intubation

- If you want intubated--for how long do you want left on the vent

- Artificially administered fluids and nutrition

    o No feeding tube

    o A trial period of feeding tube

    o Long-term feeding tube

    o No IV fluids

    o A trial of IV fluids

- Antibiotics or no antibiotics

- Future hospitalization/transfer (for long-term care residents and home patients---this is much needed)

Some of these forms also have a place for the healthcare provider to sign and date each time they review the orders with the patient. This is very important especially for those with chronic medical conditions or terminal illnesses. How often do those of us who actually have DNR orders go back and review them for any changes we may want.

You can find several links on my website where you can download each state's appropriate DNR order, MOLST, POLST, and living will forms at www.tracipowell.com .

Problem #9: Financial Benefits to Families

As sick as it may sound, you would fall over if you knew how often this issue comes into play. How many times have you read in the paper where some poor soul died and their family member didn't report it for several years? They just left the body in the house decaying so they could continue receiving that person's social security check. Well unfortunately, it's no different in medicine. We see frail elderly people who should have died years ago but the family insists that we keep doing everything possible to keep them alive while they continue to collect the patient's pension.

Have another true story for you:

I was taking care of an old man who was in very critical condition. He was on a ventilator with multiple IV cardiac drips running to keep him alive. He had three sons from a first marriage and was currently remarried to a second wife.

During the first several days that he was in ICU he could understand what we were saying to him and would nod his head appropriately to our questions. Throughout his entire stay his wife would not allow any of his three sons to come back into the room to see him. Unfortunately the law says unless you have a living will, your spouse is the person who is able to make decisions for you while you are incapacitated. This includes who gets to visit you and who does not. I will tell you right now, this is the number one problem we have with families in ICU. The decision-maker will not allow others in the family to see the patient; this is especially true when it's a blended (step-parent/step-child) family.

We informed the wife that we were doing everything possible to keep her husband alive but that he could die at any time. I remember her making frantic calls to their family lawyer wanting to get the man's will changed. One evening when she left, she came up to me and literally begged me to keep her husband alive until morning. She said she had reached her lawyer and he would be able to come into the hospital tomorrow and have the gentleman's will changed. She shared with me that her husband had a significant amount of land and currently it was to go to his sons upon his death. But she said they had talked recently and he had changed his mind and wanted her to have it all; he just hadn't got around to changing the will. …Yeah, right lady. I have to be honest here. I couldn't help but hope that the man would die before morning. It was already killing me knowing his three sons were not allowed to see their father on his deathbed, and now she was going to have them cut out of the will.

Unfortunately the patient was still alive the next day when I came back into work. When I went in to do my assessment the patient was no longer responding to any of my questions. He just laid there with his eyes half open, too weak to move. Later in the morning the wife brought a gentleman up to me who introduced himself as the patient's lawyer. He asked me if I thought the man could make an informed decision. I told him absolutely not. The lawyer asked me several more times in various ways if I thought the patient could understand what was being said to him. I repeatedly told the lawyer I had no indication that the patient could comprehend anything I was saying to him any longer. I was unable to get any response out of him the entire morning. The lawyer then wanted to know if I thought the patient would be able to sign his name. I told him I had not seen the patient lift any of his extremities in several days, so no, he was not able to sign his name.

I had heard of three similar instances in our unit during the last three to four years of other family members bringing lawyers into the ICU and having wills changed. In those other instances the lawyer had the nurse sign the papers as a witness. I made it very clear there was absolutely no way I would sign anything as a witness for this patient while he was in the condition that he was in.

The wife and lawyer proceeded to go into the patient's room. The lawyer spoke to the patient, told him who he was, and that he had revised his will and needed for him to sign it. The man made no movement. The lawyer then put a pen in the patient's hand, picked up his arm saying "Let me help you" and then 'helped' the man sign the new will.

Right after the lawyer left the wife told us to discontinue all life-support. We did. The man died within minutes.

Now our ICU is not unique. It's a 16-bed unit in a 222-bed hospital located in a small city. In the matter of just several years this type of situation happened four times. If it happens in our hospital, you better believe it happens all over the country.

Problem #10: Religious/Moral Beliefs of Families and Physicians

Hope is probably one of the most powerful emotions we humans have. When someone we love is facing death, we often cling to hope desperately. When I talk to families about the possibility of their loved one not surviving and suggest they consider a change of code status, I am often told by a spouse or adult child "God can do miracles". I then tell them that I too believe that God can do miracles, but that I know he can do miracles without all of our machines and interventions.

To put it bluntly: Hope is a great thing…but false hope is a terrible thing, costing much physically, mentally, emotionally, and financially.

I think it's a safe assumption that physicians go into medicine to save people. Look at part of the Hippocratic Oath:

I will use those dietary regimens which will benefit

my patients according to my greatest ability and judgment,

and I will do no harm or injustice to them.

I will not give a lethal drug to anyone if I am asked,

nor will I advise such a plan;…

Even though the Hippocratic Oath is rarely used in its original form today, it serves as a foundation for other similar oaths and laws that define good medical practice and morals. Such oaths are regularly taken today by medical graduates about to enter medical practice.

Here's the problem: This oath was written in the 4th century B.C. Do you know what the life expectancy was at that time?

Rome (100 to 400 BC)

Life expectancy was 22 to 30 years

Today

Life expectancy is about 78 years

Do you see the problem here? Hearts don't usually wear out at twenty-two years. Kidneys don't normally shut down at thirty years old. But in the seventh, eighth, and ninth decade of life, they often do.

Costs

As cold as it may sound, medical care is not an infinite resource. We only have so many resources to cover all of us. Let me share some numbers with you:

- Healthcare spending in 2006 totaled $2.1 trillion, or 16% of GDP

- Most healthcare dollars in the United States is spent on end-of-life care

- Medicare is the largest funding source for end-of-life care, serving more than 80 percent of people who die in the United States each year

- Approximately one-quarter of Medicare's annual budget is spent on its beneficiaries' last year of life

Many argue that because 10% to 12% of all healthcare expenditures and 27% of Medicare expenditures are spent at the end of life, and because these expenditures frequently fail to provide significant health benefits, the elimination of such care would make resources available for other unmet needs.

Not only is the government burdened with extraordinary medical expenses, so too is the patient and their families. A couple can spend a life-time acquiring a home, retirement, a few assets, and when one of them becomes critically ill even for just a short time, their entire life savings can be wiped out.

The current model guiding the delivery of healthcare in America-especially end-of-life care-is rooted in the belief that aggressive treatment is the most appropriate care strategy. The current financial incentives governing how hospitals and physicians provide care are not conducive to palliative approaches. The current payment systems are designed primarily to support acute, episodic care, rather than chronic and advanced illness.

Futile Care

Despite the growing proclivity to administer life-sustaining treatments, research indicates that increases in interventions have not reduced mortality rates. In many cases, life-sustaining treatments only prolonged the dying process.

Now I want you to go back up and read the above paragraph again. And again. And again. This is want drives nurses in critical care absolutely nuts. We have people in their eighties and nineties in ICUs everywhere who have chronic terminal illnesses, who are kept on ventilators with a tracheotomy, who have dialysis daily because their kidneys have shut down, who are long term diabetics with multiple amputations, who have a feeding tube put into their stomachs so we can keep giving them nutrition to keep them alive, and for what?! Most people will tell you they never want to be 'kept alive' on machines if there is little or no hope for a recovery back to a reasonable quality of life. Yet it happens every day.

Nurses are really good at making patients look good. We bath our patients, comb their hair back, prop them up with pillows…heck, we can make a dead person look good. What you don't see is the ulcer on the buttocks that has eaten clear through to the bone. What you don't see is all the edema (swelling), causing the man's scrotum to swell to the size of a cantaloupe. You don't see all the skin breakdown from where the patient is incontinent of stool. And you definitely don't see the pain on their faces every time we turn them or do another invasive procedure or draw labs on them for the third time that day. Many of us in critical care often ask ourselves…"Is it torture or is it care?" Daleen, a friend of mine that I use to work with, had several days straight of patients all similar to what I just described above. ..patients with chronic illnesses and advanced age who were having multiple life-sustaining but painful treatments being done. She turned to me and said "I feel like I've been a hospice nurse the last few days instead of an ICU nurse. All I've taken care of lately is people we can't save; people who I know are going to die very soon."

Another sad but true story: We had a lady in her fifties who had terminal brain cancer. Everything had been done that was possible. There was absolutely nothing else left to try. Her Power-of-Attorney (the person authorized to make her healthcare decisions) lived in Florida (we're in Ohio) and our case managers would contact this person daily regarding a change in her code status. It was explained to this POA that nothing else could be done for the patient and all we were doing was prolonging her death with lots of painful interventions. Yet the POA continued to keep the patient as a full code.

In the past, families fought to withdraw life support; now they fight to continue life support. Once again, we live in a 'lawsuit-happy' country and being named in a lawsuit, or even just threatened with one, pretty much ruins your whole day.

I was talking to a life-flight nurse one day who had worked for a children's hospital for over twenty years. We started discussing this issue of providing all this aggressive treatment on our elderly population and she said to me, "You know, at the children's hospital that I work at, children are coded for thirty minutes…maximum; neonates are coded for fifteen minutes…maximum. And yet, we'll work for hours on an eighty year old, often coding them several times throughout the day." She then went on to say, "If you give enough epi to an old piece of leather, you're going to eventually get a heartbeat." (Epi=epinephrine, the main drug we use during resuscitation) What she meant by that is yes we might get the heart to beat again but often the brain is gone, usually along with the kidneys and liver. At the children's hospital where this nurse worked, they knew if you didn't get the child back quickly, the child would be brain dead with multiple end-organ (liver, kidney) damage.

One of my favorite sayings:

"We are one of those societies that regard death as an option."

by Gail Wilensky, John M. Olin Senior Fellow at Project HOPE. Retrieved from

Financing End-of-Life Care, Challenges for An Aging Population, February 2003

So What Can We Do to Make Things Better?

For all individuals:

Complete an advance directive and living will, but most importantly, make sure you have the support of your family who will be willing to honor your wishes. And if they won't, find someone who will and take the necessary steps to make them your Power-of-Attorney. Give copies of your paperwork to all of your pertinent family members. Talk with your healthcare provider about your wishes and any questions you may have. If they won't take the time to discuss DNRs with you, find another provider. Talk with your parents, spouses, and children and find out what their wishes are in regards to end-of-life care and their desire for aggressive interventions. Trust me. If you ever have to make a decision for that person on whether or not to continue life-support, it WILL make it easier knowing what that person wanted. And if you want to make sure your assets REALLY go to the people you want to have them, talk to a lawyer. Maybe your will can be drawn up with the stipulation that it can only be changed with the approval of an outside person that you are competent to change it-a person who you name and who stands to gain nothing.

For all healthcare providers:

We need to be diligent in talking with our patients regarding what their wishes are and encouraging them to use advance directives, and even more importantly, sharing their wishes with their families. Talk to all patients of all ages, not just your elderly patients. And do it now. Don't wait until they're faced with a life or death situation.

For individuals *and* healthcare providers:

There is a great need for an increase in the use of palliative care and hospice. If prolonging death is all that is happening, let's use these more appropriate healthcare resources to care of our patients, ourselves, and our loved ones.

For the government and insurance companies:

Make big changes. Pay for preventive care. Pay for treatment of chronic illnesses. Pay better for hospice and palliative care. Hold individuals responsible for their own health in regards to smoking and obesity. Stop spending millions of dollars on futile care.

I always like the billboard signs that say 'Buckle up, it's the law'. It's short and to the point. Why not a national campaign about advance directives? There is an absolutely fabulous advertisement I've seen on TV about smoking. It starts out with cool shots of people smoking but then ends with an older man, bald, thin, naked, sitting in a wheelchair in a solid white room with an IV and oxygen on who looks like he's dying of lung cancer, and he says something like 'Smoking isn't as great as it looks'. Now THAT'S A GREAT commercial! I rarely watch TV but one viewing of that commercial and it has stayed with me. Why not do a commercial showing some elderly person with multiple IVs, on a ventilator with a tracheotomy, a Foley catheter in their bladder, a rectal tube, a peg tube going into their stomach, malnourished, and one leg amputated with a nurse standing at the bedside asking "Is this torture or is this care?"

My contribution: This book.

I realize that parts of this book will make some people uncomfortable. It will probably make some people angry. That is not my intention. I believe a patient should be a partner with their healthcare provider. My goal for this book is to simply try to educate the public so they can make informed decisions about their care and perhaps be a little better prepared for a difficult journey we must all travel—the ending of our life on this great earth.

Two out of three people

die in hospitals or

nursing homes

Final Thoughts

I was finished with my book with the previous page. Then my husband Paul proofread my book for me and said I needed to "soften" things up in closing, to give people hope. Being a wife *and* nurse, I started ranting that the purpose of my book was to give people facts, not be all warm and fuzzy. But my husband (who hates hospitals, doctors, anything medical) is a wise man when it comes to life and he explained to me that I need to let the public know that everyone has a right to die with dignity. He said you have these people who have lived for a very long time, who have always been independent, who are very proud people, and they could end up lying somewhere with all kinds of tubes stuck in them and not be able to do anything for themselves. Paul said let them know they are entitled to die with dignity.

Once again in our many years of marriage…he is right. Death is part of life. It does not have to be feared. Some people talk of a 'peaceful death' or a 'good death'. Being at home, surrounded by people you love, pain free, and at peace in your soul. That sounds like a good death. A peaceful death. A death with dignity. You do have a RIGHT to that.

LIVE

WELL

Works Cited

(2008). Retrieved November 21, 2008, from Oath of Hippocrates: www.cirp.org

(2008). Retrieved January 4, 2009, from Ohio Department of Health.

(2008). Retrieved October 16, 2008, from Compassion and Support - Professionals: www.compassionandsupport.org

Austin, B., & Fleisher, L. (2003). *Financing End-of-Life Care.* The Robert Wood Johnson Foundation.

Benoit, M. (2008, May). The Phenomenon of Moral Distress Among Intensive Care Nurses. *American Journal of Critical Care* , p. 291.

Chind, M. (2006, May 16). 80-year-old'd chest tattoo: Do Not Resuscitate. Des Moines, Iowa.

Gibbs, N. (2008, May 5). The Light of Death. *Time* , p. 56.

Handy, C., Sulmasym, D., Merkel, C., & Ury, W. (2008). The surrogate's experience in authorizing a do not resuscitate order. *Palliative and Supportive Care* , pp. 13-19.

Lazzarini, Z., Arons, S., & Wisniewski, A. (2006). Legal and policy lessions from the Schiavo casde: Is our right to choose the medical care we want seriously at risk? *Palliative and Supportive Care* , 145-153.

Lemiengre, J., Dierckx de Casterle, B., Van Craen, K., Schotsmans, P., & Gastmans, C. (2007). Institutional ethics policies on medical end-of-life decisions: A literature review. *Science Direct* , 131-143.

Sulmasy, D., Sood, J., Texiera, K., McAuley, R., McGugins, J., & Ury, W. (2006, January 16). *A Prospective Trial of a New Policy Eliminating Signed Consent for Do Not Resuscitate Orders.* Retrieved October 10, 2008, from www.pubmedcentral.nih.gov

Thelen, M. (2005, December 25). End-Of-Life Decision Making in Intensive Care. *Critical Care Nurse* , pp. 28-37.

Wilkinson, A., Wenger, N., & Shugarman, L. (2007, June). *U.S. Department of Health and Human Serivces.* Retrieved October 3, 2008, from Literature Review on Advance Directives: www.aspe.hhs.gov

www.ingramcontent.com/pod-product-compliance
Lightning Source LLC
Chambersburg PA
CBHW052008280526
45793CB00005B/902